NIGHT BRILLIANCE

The Sleep Thinker's Guide to Powerful Problem-Solving

Praise for the sleep thinking process and for *Night Brilliance*

"This is a journal and a process definitely worth the investment of time and practice for those seeking to live with more peace, awareness, creativity and ease."
—EMMA RAE RHEAD, M.D., hyphnotherapist and coach

"Sleep thinking is a subtle practice, and the journal makes space for meaningful questions to take root. Though I am early in my sleep thinking journey, I already appreciate the shift in how I think about sleep and problem-solving. I sense something meaningful unfolding beneath the surface. The sleep thinking journal has helped me approach my nights with more intention and trust—it's a simple practice that feels rich with possibility."—KELLY GAMMON, healthcare and higher education IT Specalist

"I've been using for about fifteen days now and I love it! This has been so helpful in giving me a greater understanding of the process—not just an intellectual understanding, but actual practice with the process. The journal makes it so easy! It reminds me that I can tap into this unexplored resource and rich and expansive process. It's all about participating with something already going on inside me in new and rewarding ways. That's been so helpful!"—ELLE GARFIELD, awareness couselor

"After sleep thinking for a couple of nights, an entire flow of ideas started to come through. These ideas were much lighter and more colorful than my conscious, trying-hard brain typically produces. I'm a big proponent of 'sleeping on it' and often delay a decision that is not clear to me. However, I hadn't previously considered making sleep thinking a more consistent practice. Now I will. I think this will help nagging problems no longer nag!"
—KIRSTEN JOHANSEN, executive coach

"The adage 'sleep on it' takes on a whole new meaning with Eric Maisel's sleep thinking journal. When I followed Maisel's encouraging prompts and practiced my own pre-sleep questions, I felt permission to trust my sleep thinking. The strategy to wonder and tap into my 'committee of sleep' helped me relax; and upon waking, I was able to approach my regular daytime worries with more ease. This practice has even helped me access creative alternatives to challenges and negative self-talk during my waking hours!"—MUIREANN O'CALLAGHAN, writing coach and mentor

"After just one week of use, I received great insights and made great progress in my chosen areas. I'm excited about the possibilities that sleep thinking holds!"
—MARK RIDOUT, international touring jazz musician

"After just a few days of using the sleep thinking program, I started to notice that I was getting answers to my questions. I'm not sure how that happened, but I'm sure enough receiving answers, downloads, and direction!"
—PAMELA WRIGHT, certified life coach

"Sleep thinking—what a wonderful tool! I've gotten answers in my sleep before but never added prompts with journaling. I found by practicing, I was much clearer on my projects and how to approach things in my waking hours. I would wake up excited to have answers to my questions and often had a clear vision of what needed to be done. This results in less stress for me. Thank you for sharing this tool with me!!!"—PAT HOUSE, visual artist

"In his sleep thinking journal, Eric Maisel helps us explore the idea that the sleeping brain isn't just for random dreaming. Through questions and prompts, Maisel helps us prepare our brains to solve problems and answer questions while we sleep. With patience and persistence, we can train our brains to focus on a question, and then be ready for the answer. This process can even help in dealing with anxieties and sleep issues, by turning them consciously over to the brain to work on while we sleep. A guide for seekers, creatives, and anyone who wants to better utilize their brain's potential, this is a valuable addition to any journaling or meditation practice."
—JANA VAN DER VEER, book coach

"Eric Maisel offers a revolutionary yet elegantly simple method: harnessing "sleep thinking" to work through challenges you might otherwise wrestle with for days or weeks. The approach is refreshingly uncomplicated and accessible: Each chapter provides a straightforward question to ponder and journal about, along with a single prompt before bedtime. You then allow your brain to work while you sleep, and welcome the insights in the morning through journaling. What sets this guide apart is its combination of inspiring insight and real-world usability. Maisel invites readers not just to dream, but to think purposefully while asleep and then make room to receive and act on the answers that emerge. It's a fresh way to tap into your subconscious mind, all while gaining rest!"
—JULIANA BRUNO, author of Reasons to Live

NIGHT BRILLIANCE

The Sleep Thinker's Guide to Powerful Problem-Solving

ERIC MAISEL, PhD

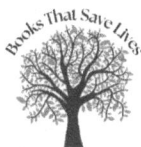

Books That Save Lives

Published by BTSL/Jim Dandy Publishing
6252 Peach Avenue
Van Nuys, CA 91411
info@jimdandypublishing.com

For bulk orders, special quantities, course adoptions, and corporate
sales, please email info@jimdandypublishing.com

ISBN: 978-1-96366-731-8
BISAC: MEDICAL / Sleep Medicine MED119000

For Ann, forty-eight years into this adventure

Table of Contents

Introduction

Imagine acquiring an amazing problem-solving tool that takes absolutely no extra time, that produces fantastic results, and that is as free as free can be. That's what I'm offering!

That you haven't heard much about this tool, or maybe even anything, is a shame. This was always available to you, as it is part of your native inheritance as a human being. It's a shame if you haven't been using sleep thinking to increase your creativity, solve your problems, and reduce your stress. But it's still available to you, so let's get you using it!

When you sleep, you dream. That you know already. Everybody knows about our ability to dream. But very few people seem to know that when we sleep, we also think. Not dream, think!

It's easy not to clearly hear this distinction. People are so accustomed to associating "sleep" with "dreaming" that they have trouble getting this important distinction. But we don't just dream when we sleep. We also think!

What do I mean by "think?" Exactly what you take "think" to mean. Solving a math problem is a "thinking" sort of thing. Trying to rationally decide between two hard choices is a "thinking" sort of thing. Wondering what business task to tackle next is a "thinking" sort of thing. Using clues to solve a mystery is a "thinking" sort of thing. You get the idea!

We try to sleep, but our brain keeps percolating. That's why it can keep us awake at night, because it is still busily doing its thing, maybe worrying about something, maybe replaying an event of the day, maybe rehearsing an interaction that's coming up tomorrow. Our brain, as we try to get to sleep, can do a lot of fretting.

Fretting like this can keep us awake—and does keep us awake so often (and so persistently) that, as a nation and as a world, we're experiencing a real insomnia epidemic. This unproductive thinking—all this fearful worrying and uncontrolled obsessing—is the brain thinking, but not in ways that serve us. The thinking I'm talking about is very different from that! I'm talking about positive, productive thinking, really our very best thinking.

Even when we do fall asleep, our brain still stays busy. It generates dreams, as you know. But it will also think—about whatever you invite it to think about. And it will think beautifully and richly, often better than your awake thinking. Often much better. That's the thinking we're after!

Why better? Because, during the day, we get distracted by this and that. Maybe we're obliged to deal with a noisy environment, or with interruptions. Maybe we're in the habit of trying to think while also doing something else. And so on. To put it one way, when we're awake, we only use a portion of our brain—only a portion of our native inheritance. When we're asleep, we have our whole brain available! Isn't that good to know?

But how can you make use of this sleep thinking if, well, you're asleep? Are you obliged to wake up and "grab" what you were just thinking? Not at all. The answer is really very simple. All you need to do is the following. Before you go to sleep, aim your brain in the direction you want it to go by asking it a "sleep thinking question" or by providing it with a "sleep thinking prompt." Then let your brain do its thing.

Next comes a crucial step—when you wake up, you "process the night" by holding yourself open to receiving what your brain would like to provide. You start each new day not with a bagel, yoga, or meditation, but by holding yourself open to receive what your brain has worked out during the night. It has information to provide you! Answers are there. But you must make space for them. This is simplicity itself. And it is the very opposite of work!

Take the following example. You are writing a novel. You have a pivotal scene coming up between Mary and John. This is a "big deal" scene and you want to get it right. So you've been kind of avoiding trying to write it. That is often what we do, especially if life is busy and distracting.

What to do? The beautiful, wise, and simple thing to do is to invite your sleeping brain to write the scene. You do this by going to bed with a "wonder" that aims your brain in the direction that you desire it to go. This "wonder" might sound like, "I wonder what Mary wants to say to John when they get back from the party."

Your brain is entirely likely to take your invitation to heart and create exactly the scene you need. Are you guaranteed the perfect scene, or even any scene at all? Sadly, no. Answers take as long as they take, and you can't really rush them. But, on the other hand, your brain might deliver you that vital scene that very night! Often it will.

But it will deliver it only if you are open to receiving it. What does this particular openness look like? It looks like you heading to your computer, with maybe a brief stop at the bathroom and at the kitchen for coffee, turning on your computer, and murmuring, "Now, what was it that Mary wanted to say to John?" That's it!

It is quite possible that all you would need to do is take dictation, as your brain delivers you the scene it created in the middle of the night.

Take a moment and consider that scenario. Rather than having to fuss about that pivotal scene, rather than worrying about that scene, rather than avoiding writing that scene, rather than having your novel stall because you've been avoiding that scene, you would, without any heavy lifting whatsoever, have had that scene delivered right to you. Can you imagine any home delivery service better than that?

Each of the following two-page spreads provides you with the opportunity to consider some aspect of sleep thinking, journal on that idea, create a sleep thinking prompt, use that sleep thinking prompt to orient your brain that night, and then process your sleep thinking in the morning. Let's get started! Your sleep thinking adventure awaits you.

Note:

This journal is organized as seventy-five invitations. But there is no need to follow this scheme in a linear way, as some of the ideas or themes may not resonate for you or pertain to you.

Once you get the hang of sleep thinking, which may happen as soon as the first night, please feel free to use this journal as an aid to clarify the sleep thinking process and as a resource to provoke your thinking.

You might follow this journal prompt by prompt and idea by idea. That is certainly a rich way to proceed! But you can also dip into it, jump around, and make use of it in your own way. Either way, you will be amazed at what your brain can do—while you are getting a good night's sleep!

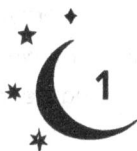

THE MOTHER OF THOUGHTS

"Night is the mother of thoughts."
—JOHN FLORIO

We think while we sleep. That makes our sleeping brain one of our greatest problem-solving tools. It thinks uninvited, and it also thinks invited. It serves us best when we invite it to think, for instance when we invite it to solve a problem that's puzzling us, point us toward the next step in life, or provide us with a plan for recovery or growth.

Do a little journaling using the following journal prompt: "Can I remember times when my sleeping brain did some good thinking that served me well?"

_____

_____

_____

_____

_____

From your journaling, arrive at a sleep thinking prompt—that is, at the instruction you want to provide your brain about where it should focus its thinking while you sleep. Arrive at your own, or use the following sleep thinking prompt to get started.

Sleep Thinking Prompt: "Tonight is my first night consciously employing my sleep thinking. I'm going to ask my brain to think about the following problem that's bothering me."

Then, in the morning, as soon as you awake, turn directly to processing the night by writing in this journal. You might repeat your sleep thinking prompt, or ask yourself a question like, "What have I learned?" or "What would my brain like to provide me?"

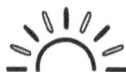

_____

_____

_____

_____

_____

Morning Processing:

_____

_____

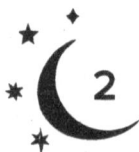

LET ME SLEEP ON IT

" 'Let me sleep on it' is not always a way of
postponing a decision. It may also be a recourse
to the folk wisdom that knows that there is more
than one way to think about a problem."
—A. ALVAREZ

We all know the phrase "Sleep on it." That innocent-sounding phrase captures a brilliant truth about our brain, that it consolidates thoughts, creates, problem-solves, and works wonderfully efficiently while we sleep.

Journal Prompt: "What does the phrase 'sleep on it' mean to me?"

_____

_____

_____

_____

_____

Sleep Thinking Prompt: "I wonder what it wouldbe like to 'sleep on' problems, rather than to struggle to solve them with my overworked daytime brain."

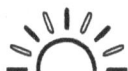

_____

_____

_____

_____

Morning Processing:

_____

_____

_____

_____

_____

_____

_____

_____

_____

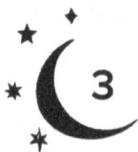

WAKING NECESSITIES

"A waking man, being under the necessity of having some ideas constantly, is not at liberty to think."
—JOHN LOCKE

When we're awake, too much occupies us for us to think at our best. With text messages, errands, worries about the kids and our finances, making sure to check twice before crossing the road, remembering to pay our taxes or pick up eggs at the market...how much of our brain is left to work on the novel we're writing, or to think carefully about that vexing inheritance dispute with our brother? Not enough, usually.

Journal Prompt: "What is my experience of trying to do good, solid thinking during an ordinary vexing, taxing day like?"

_____

_____

_____

_____

Sleep Thinking Prompt: "I wonder what it would be like if I used my nights rather than my days to solve my problems. Would my days benefit if I engaged in sleep thinking?"

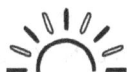

_____

_____

_____

_____

Morning Processing:

_____

_____

_____

_____

_____

_____

_____

_____

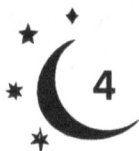

THE BEAUTY OF OBLIVION

"In descending stage 1 of NREM sleep, soon either we are utterly oblivious or we enter a most peculiar sleep-thought mode."
—J. ALLAN HOBSON

During the day, we stand ready for what comes next. We are obliged to be alert and awake. At night, we allow ourselves to enter the most blissful oblivion. Not only does sleep thinking help us solve problems, reduce our stress, and increase our creativity, it occurs without our presence, as it were, as we engage in the most wonderful vanishing act our species has been granted—sleep. Embrace, rather than fear, that oblivion.

Journal Prompt: "Waking is alertness. Sleep is oblivion. Do I relish that oblivion...or do I maybe fear it?"

_____

_____

_____

Sleep Thinking Prompt: "I wonder what might want to emerge tonight in the wonderful oblivion that is deep sleep."

_____

_____

_____

Morning Processing:

_____

_____

_____

_____

_____

_____

_____

_____

_____

5

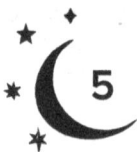

MUCH TOO ECONOMICAL

*"Nature is much too economical to waste
hours of biological time doing nothing but
saving energy and idling the brain."*
—J. ALLAN HOBSON

The beauty of sleep thinking is that it is the very opposite of wasting time. We waste time in so many ways: getting stuck in traffic, falling down some internet rabbit hole, doing tasks that we don't love but that must get done, and so on. But nature has generously given us one splendid way not to waste time. It has given us the chance to do some excellent thinking and creating while we sleep. Let's not waste that opportunity!

Journal Prompt: "What would it be like to acquire the habit of sleep thinking as a way to make great, efficient use of my time?"

_____

_____

_____

Sleep Thinking Prompt: "Tonight, I would like to make lovely, efficient use of my sleep thinking time to ponder the following:"

_____

_____

_____

Morning Processing:

_____

_____

_____

_____

_____

_____

_____

_____

_____

_____

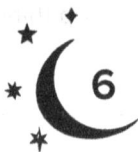

THE QUIET CLASSROOM

"Dreaming is often a theater of emotion and image;
sleep thinking is more like a quiet classroom
where the mind whispers its reflections."
—ANONYMOUS

Remember that we are talking about thinking and not about dreaming. Dreams are wonderful, memorable, and useful in their own way. But we are talking about thinking, not dreaming. Thinking is a second thing your brain can and does do while you sleep. It is the difference between the brain dreaming up a lovely story set in outer space and the brain arriving at an understanding of the exact relationship between mass and energy. Yes, the two can weave together, and answers may come as dream images. But let's keep our eye on the distinction between dreaming and thinking. It's an important one!

Journal Prompt: "What do I sense as the differences between dreaming and thinking?"

_____

_____

_____

_____

Sleep Thinking Prompt: "I wonder what it would be like to have a dream tonight that also solves a problem. Might my brain like to marry dreaming and thinking?"

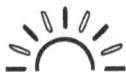

_____

_____

_____

_____

Morning Processing:

_____

_____

_____

_____

_____

_____

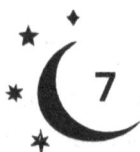

MORE THAN OURSELVES

"We are more than ourselves in our sleep."
—THOMAS BROWNE

Very often, we feel less than ourselves. We have the feeling that we aren't using our full capabilities or really manifesting our potential. What would it feel like to be at our best and use every ounce of our capabilities? That's the way what goes on as we sleep can feel! Free of necessity, free to go back or forward in time, free to think about anything and everything, we can finally feel as large as we are. This is a dramatic benefit of sleep thinking, that it gives us the chance to experience ourselves at our best and brightest.

Journal Prompt: "What would it feel like to be at my best?"

_____

_____

_____

_____

Sleep Thinking Prompt: "I wonder what might want to emerge if I suggest to my brain that it sleep think 'me at my best'.

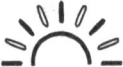

_____

_____

_____

_____

Morning Processing:

_____

_____

_____

_____

_____

_____

_____

_____

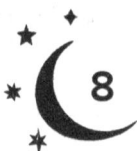

OUR RICHLY COLORED NIGHT

*"I often think that the night is more alive
and richly colored than the day."*
—VINCENT VAN GOGH

What can prevent us from reaping the benefits of sleep thinking? One obstacle might be our very relationship to sleep, to darkness, and to the night. We may have a troubled relationship with darkness, and maybe even fear it. Rather than night and sleep feeling alive in a good sense, it may feel alive in a bad sense: as a place of threats and nightmares. What sort of relationship do you have with darkness, the night, and sleep?

Journal Prompt: "What is my relationship with darkness, the night, and sleep?"

_____

_____

_____

_____

Sleep Thinking Prompt: "I wonder what it would be like to feel completely safe and at ease as I sleep tonight."

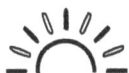

_____

_____

_____

_____

Morning Processing:

_____

_____

_____

_____

_____

_____

_____

_____

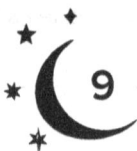

THE BETTER HALF OF LIFE

"Night is the other half of life, and the better half."
—GOETHE

Let us begin to affirm that sleep is, if not the better half of life, certainly not the worst half. Let us give it its due and begin to honor its value and its important place in our life. It is restorative; it is full of liveliness; it hugs us and comforts us. And it is the place where we do our best thinking. Might it be time to give sleep its due?

Journal Prompt: "What would it be like if I began to picture sleep as 'the better half of life'?"

_____

_____

_____

_____

_____

Sleep Thinking Prompt: "I wonder what it would be like to really enjoy sleep."

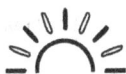

_____

_____

_____

_____

Morning Processing:

_____

_____

_____

_____

_____

_____

_____

_____

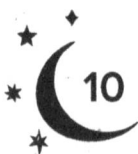

OH, THOUGHTFUL NIGHT!

"Oh, huge and thoughtful night!"
—WALT WHITMAN

Our sleep thinking can be brilliant and encompassing. During the day, as we work on a problem, we may find ourselves trapped in minutiae or stuck in a dead-end corner. When we sleep, we expand. We can see the whole picture, even if that picture is huge. We can travel faster than the speed of light and get to the edge of the universe in nanoseconds. Wouldn't this get you better answers than if you stayed small and played small, as we tend to do during the day?

Journal Prompt: "What would it be like to get bigger, better answers to the problems I face and to the puzzles I try to solve?"

_____

_____

_____

_____

Sleep Thinking Prompt: "I wonder, brain, if you would like to provide me with something huge tonight."

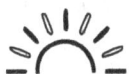

_____

_____

_____

_____

Morning Processing:

_____

_____

_____

_____

_____

_____

_____

_____

_____

11

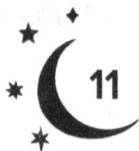

WIDER THAN THE SKY

"The brain is wider than the sky."
—EMILY DICKINSON

Maybe thinking makes you a little anxious. Maybe you're often tired of your usual thoughts. Maybe your brain seems to rush off without your consent. Let's start fresh tonight. With loving kindness, but also with some firmness, enter into a new, better relationship with your brain, one that welcomes your brain's brilliance. What might that new relationship look like?

Journal Prompt: "I can picture myself entering into a new relationship with my brain. I think that might look like the following."

_____

_____

_____

_____

Sleep Thinking Prompt: "I wonder what it would be like to have a whole new relationship with my brain."

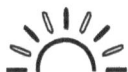

_____

_____

_____

_____

Morning Processing:

_____

_____

_____

_____

_____

_____

_____

_____

12

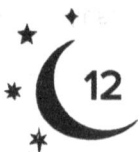

CONFIDENT SLEEP

*"You know, sleep and confidence
are almost the same thing."*
—UGO BETTI

Tens of millions of people have a troubled relationship with sleep. They find it hard to get to sleep, they toss and turn, they're susceptible to nightmares, they wake up abruptly and find it hard—even impossible—to get back to sleep. And they envy those who sleep peacefully. Let's begin the road back to peaceful sleep. Wouldn't it be lovely to go to bed confident of a good night's sleep?"

Journal Prompt: "I know that my relationship with sleep could be better. By that, I think I mean the following."

_____

_____

_____

_____

Sleep Thinking Prompt: "I wonder what it would be like to learn why my sleep is so troubled."

_____

_____

_____

_____

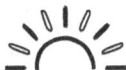

Morning Processing:

_____

_____

_____

_____

_____

_____

_____

_____

_____

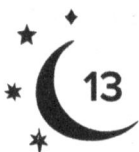

FREE-REIN SLEEP

"Researchers suggest that novel solutions are possible in sleep because we give our thoughts and images free rein without distractions from the environment."
—JAMES B. HAAS

During the day, you're likely holding the reins tight on your life. You aim for control, because you know what can happen if you lose control. But maybe you can surrender when you sleep? Maybe you let go of the reins then? Maybe you can provide yourself with permission to let whatever wants to come come?

Journal Prompt: "I think I still try to maintain control of my thoughts and feelings while I sleep for the following reasons."

_____

_____

_____

_____

Sleep Thinking Prompt: "I wonder what it would be like to give my brain free rein tonight."

_____

_____

_____

_____

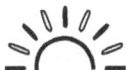

Morning Processing:

_____

_____

_____

_____

_____

_____

_____

_____

_____

14

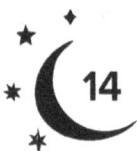

THINKING HARDER

"We often find the answer not by thinking harder,
but by letting go—and sleep helps us let go."
—DAVID EAGLEMAN

Remember not knowing the answer to a question on a test and trying to "think harder," hoping that "thinking harder" would get you the answer? How often did it work? Probably not very often. Sleep thinking is the very opposite approach. You offer yourself a sleep thinking prompt as you go to sleep, and then you let go. No holding tight, no thinking harder. Just surrender.

Journal Prompt: "I am not very good at surrendering. I think this might be the case because of the following."

_____

_____

_____

_____

Sleep Thinking Prompt: "I wonder what would emerge if I relaxed my brain and surrendered to the night."

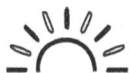

_____

_____

_____

_____

Morning Processing:

_____

_____

_____

_____

_____

_____

_____

_____

_____

15

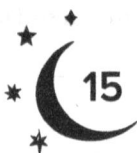

WE ARE NOT HYPOCRITES

"We are not hypocrites in our sleep."
—WILLIAM HAZLITT

Human beings are well-known to be defensive creatures. We deny unpleasant truths, rationalize away our mistakes, project onto others what we ourselves are feeling, and so on. But when we sleep, our sleeping brain sloughs off much of its defensiveness. We are, as Hazlitt puts it, not hypocrites in our sleep. Rather, we are our most authentic selves. Isn't that a relief? Mustn't that reduce a great deal of our stress, to relax into our truth which, as the old adage has it, sets us free?

Journal Prompt: "I think my defensiveness manifests in the following ways."

_____

_____

_____

_____

Sleep Thinking Prompt: "I wonder what it would feel like to defend myself less. Might that even reduce my stress levels?"

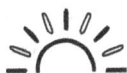

_____

_____

_____

_____

Morning Processing:

_____

_____

_____

_____

_____

_____

_____

_____

_____

16

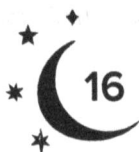

A WORLD OF OUR OWN

"All men whilst they are awake are in one common world. But each of them, when he is asleep, is in a world of his own."
—PLUTARCH

It can prove a struggle to retain our individuality in the face of life's demands that we fit in, not make waves, obey the rules, and go along to get along. When we're awake, all that pressure to conform presses in on us. But when we sleep, we can sleep-think worlds of our own. Whether we dream them into existence or think them into existence, those unique, personal worlds are available to us when we sleep. Sleep is one place to be the person you really are.

Journal Prompt: "It has been a lifelong struggle to retain my individuality and independence. Sleep thinking can help in this regard in the following ways."

_____

_____

_____

Sleep Thinking Prompt: "I wonder what it would be like for me to be completely me while I sleep."

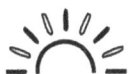

_____

_____

_____

_____

Morning Processing:

_____

_____

_____

_____

_____

_____

_____

_____

_____

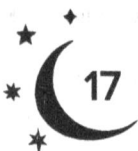

SLEEP THINKING RESPONSIBILITY

"In dreams begins responsibility."
—WILLIAM BUTLER YEATS

It is a feature of our species to not want to take responsibility. Blaming others, scapegoating others, excusing ourselves, rationalizing away our lack of effort: We are all guilty. While awake, we are habituated to avoid responsibility. But when we sleep, we can invite our sleeping brain to own up to its responsibilities. We can inch our way toward being our best self by sleep thinking in that direction. That is a wise and painless way to own up to life.

Journal Prompt: "I can see sleep thinking helping me live a more intentional, responsible life in the following ways."

_____

_____

_____

_____

Sleep Thinking Prompt: "I wonder what it would be like to invite my brain to 'take responsibility'."

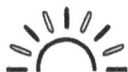

_____

_____

_____

_____

Morning Processing:

_____

_____

_____

_____

_____

_____

_____

_____

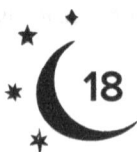

18

DAY WORK

"Creative dreams come to people who are intensely
focused on their work. Dreams do their best
when you are doing your best, in your conscious
life, to work on your problem yourself."
—HENRY REED

Sleep thinking is like that also. It is less likely that you will solve your problems or come up with creative solutions using sleep thinking unless you're also working on those problems while you're awake. It isn't a good policy to avoid a problem during the day, hoping to solve it at night. If something matters to you, it is wise that you pay attention to it waking and sleeping.

Journal Prompt: "A good plan to help me focus on my intentions would be the following."

_____

_____

_____

Sleep Thinking Prompt: "I wonder if I can return tonight to the work I've been avoiding while awake."

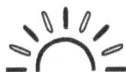

_____

_____

_____

_____

Morning Processing:

_____

_____

_____

_____

_____

_____

_____

_____

19

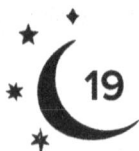

COLLABORATIONS WITH
THE UNIVERSE

*"Even sleepers are workers and collaborators
in what goes on in the universe."*
—HERACLITUS

Even the most diehard skeptic and secularist has a bit of a taste for mystery and some suspicion that more is going on in the universe than meets the eye. Is it possible that when we sleep, we collaborate with the universe? That is surely a fanciful idea; but is it maybe also a beautiful one? If you are looking for more connection with unseen worlds, isn't sleep a logical place to look?

Journal Prompt: "I think it is possible that in sleep I collaborate with the universe. By that I mean the following."

_____

_____

_____

Sleep Thinking Prompt: "I wonder what collaborations I'll enter into tonight."

_____

_____

_____

Morning Processing:

_____

_____

_____

_____

_____

_____

_____

_____

_____

_____

20

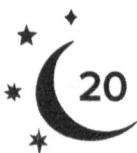

WHERE TO START?

"You don't have to see the whole staircase, just take the first step."
—MARTIN LUTHER KING, JR.

If you intend to start sleep thinking, where should you start? The starting place is deciding where you want to point your nighttime brain. What pressing issue do you want to discuss with yourself? What problem do you want to solve? What's bothering you? What do you need next: a new creative project, a business problem solved, a relationship issue tackled? Brainstorm a list of your current challenges—and then pick one to sleep think on.

Journal Prompt: "Here are the things that are currently 'up' for me."

_____

_____

_____

_____

Sleep Thinking Prompt: "Tonight I begin. I wonder what it will be like to invite my brain to sleep think. I'm excited!"

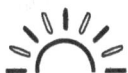

_____

_____

_____

_____

Morning Processing:

_____

_____

_____

_____

_____

_____

_____

_____

_____

21

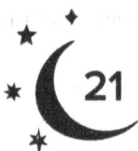

CONSCIOUS EXPLORATION

"I think that wholeness comes from living your life consciously during the day and then exploring your inner life at night."
—MARGERY CUYLER

You've fashioned a sleep thinking prompt and you offer it up to yourself. That might sound like, "I wonder how the next movement of my symphony should start," or "I wonder if I should talk to Mark about his grades." Now, what should follow in the moments before sleep? A deep surrender to the night and a deep desire to sleep think. In words, this might sound like, "I am peaceful, calm, and ready to explore."

Journal Prompt: "I understand the importance of holding an intention. Let me journal on the intention, 'I want to sleep think.' "

_____

_____

_____

Sleep Thinking Prompt: "I wonder what explorations I'm in store for tonight."

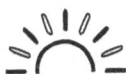

_____

_____

_____

_____

Morning Processing:

_____

_____

_____

_____

_____

_____

_____

_____

_____

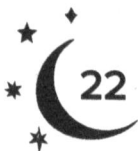

VAGUE DAYS, LOGICAL CONCLUSIONS

"Sleep seems to hammer out for me the logical conclusions of my vague days."
—D. H. LAWRENCE

You're ready to sleep. You've said your sleep thinking prompt, silently or aloud, and invited your brain to sleep think. But then some stray thought invades your mind—maybe a thought about an argument you had at work, or a presentation you have to give tomorrow. So much for sleep thinking! But wait. Calm yourself, say no to that invasive thought, and repeat your sleep thinking prompt. In short, try again. You want what your brain can provide: Don't short-circuit the process by allowing some vague thought to hijack your mind.

Journal Prompt: "I think I'll be able to return to my sleep thinking prompt, when and if an unhelpful thought intrudes, if I just remember to do the following."

_____

_____

_____

_____

Sleep Thinking Prompt: "I wonder what it would be like to only think thoughts that serve me."

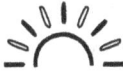

_____

_____

_____

_____

Morning Processing:

_____

_____

_____

_____

_____

_____

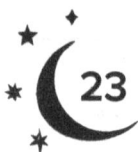

YOUR THOUGHTS
AND AFFECTIONS

"Those things that have occupied a man's thoughts and affections while awake recur to his imagination while asleep."
—THOMAS AQUINAS

Maybe you aren't certain which problem or issue you ought to focus on. Maybe so many disturbing things are going on in your life that you feel overwhelmed and incapable of choosing one place to focus. Relax. Any way in is a way in, and every solution is valuable. Just calmly notice what's occupying your waking thoughts; pick one challenge, problem, or worry from among the very many; and construct your sleep thinking prompt. Then ease yourself into the night. Tomorrow you can tackle something else. Let tonight be for this adventure.

Journal Prompt: "I will use the following process to decide which issue I'll turn over to my sleep thinking brain."

_____

_____

_____

_____

Sleep Thinking Prompt: "I'm thrilled to be working on exactly this tonight."

_____

_____

_____

_____

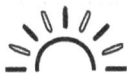

Morning Processing:

_____

_____

_____

_____

_____

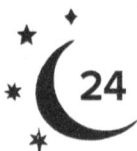

WHAT YOU CHOOSE TO FOCUS ON

"What you choose to focus on determines the quality of your life."
—SADHGURU

Once you determine what issue, problem, or challenge you intend to focus on, you will want to double-check to make sure that you've identified the issue correctly. For instance, a problem you're having with writing your memoir may actually be a problem you're having with your mate, who keeps interrupting you as you try to write. A problem you're having at home may be the residue of a problem you're having at work. Etcetera. Think carefully, and make sure that you've named your problem as accurately as you can.

Journal Prompt: "Are there other, maybe more accurate ways of thinking about the problem I've named?"

_____

_____

_____

Sleep Thinking Prompt: "I wonder if my sleeping brain might like to reframe the matter I've handed it."

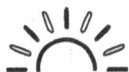

_____

_____

_____

_____

Morning Processing:

_____

_____

_____

_____

_____

_____

_____

_____

25

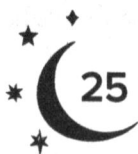

ANXIOUS BEDTIME

*"The worst thing in the world is to
try to sleep and not to."*
—F. SCOTT FITZGERALD

Anxiety gets in the way of so much in life. It may prevent you
from flying, from performing, from speaking up, from tackling
creative work, from getting a medical check-up. And from
sleep thinking. If you go to bed anxious, more with worries
than with wonders, you're more likely to get anxiety dreams
(or nightmares) than sleep thinking results. Consider the
importance of a calm entry into the night. This might even
be a place to focus your sleep thinking.

Journal Prompt: "I know that anxiety is a problem for me.
It manifests in the following ways."

_____

_____

_____

_____

Sleep Thinking Prompt: "I wonder what it would be like to go to bed more peacefully and calmly."

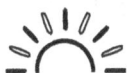

_____

_____

_____

_____

Morning Processing:

_____

_____

_____

_____

_____

_____

_____

_____

26

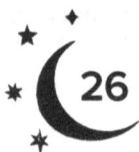

BACKGROUND ANXIETY

"Anxiety is there. It is only sleeping."
—MARTIN HEIDEGGER

Maybe you've tried to deal with your anxiety through medication, meditation, cognitive therapy, yoga, or in some other way. Give sleep thinking a try. Invite your sleeping brain to come up with a novel way to reframe your anxiety, to manage your anxiety, to heal a wound causing the anxiety, to visualize a changed, calmer you, etc. It will be happy to take on the task!

Journal Prompt: "So far, I've tried the following strategies for dealing with my anxieties."

_____

_____

_____

_____

_____

Sleep Thinking Prompt: "I wonder what it would be like to be a changed person, one who is rarely anxious?"

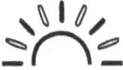

_____

_____

_____

_____

Morning Processing:

_____

_____

_____

_____

_____

_____

_____

_____

27

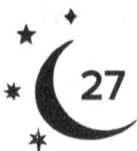

BEDTIME ROUTINES

*"I love sleep. My life has the tendency to fall
apart when I'm awake, you know?"*
—ERNEST HEMINGWAY

Even if you love to sleep, your bedtime routines may not be serving either your sleep or your sleep thinking. Staying up too late to the point of exhaustion, drinking too much alcohol, watching disturbing movies, obsessing about an event that occurred that day, checking in on world news, getting into an argument with your partner—none of this is conducive to a restful night's sleep, or to fruitful sleep thinking. What would be your perfect pre-sleep routine? And how might you acquire that perfect routine?

Journal Prompt: "I think my best bedtime routine would be the following."

_____

_____

_____

Sleep Thinking Prompt: "I wonder what my ideal bedtime routine might look like."

_____

_____

_____

_____

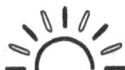

Morning Processing:

_____

_____

_____

_____

_____

_____

_____

_____

28

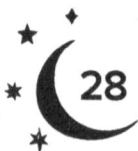

CAREFUL PROMPTING

*"One of the most adventurous things
left us is to go to bed."*
—E. V. LUCAS

You will want to take care with the exact wording of your sleep thinking prompt or question. One word might send you in one direction, and a different word might send you in a very different direction. Consider the difference between, "I wonder what I want to say to John" and "I wonder what I want from John." Wouldn't each of those prompts lead to quite different sleep thinking adventures?

Journal Prompt: "I can see the value in being really careful in how I frame my sleep thinking prompts."

_____

_____

_____

_____

Sleep Thinking Prompt: "I wonder if the way I've framed my sleep thinking prompt is on-target."

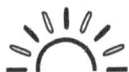

_____

_____

_____

_____

Morning Processing:

_____

_____

_____

_____

_____

_____

_____

_____

29

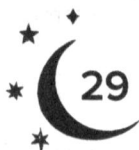

INVITING CHANGE

"Asking questions is the first way to begin to change."
—KUBRA SAIT

Your sleep thinking prompt is an invitation. You are inviting your brain to provide you with information, but you are also inviting change. Between the lines, you are saying, "I need answers, even if they are painful, even if they make work for me, and even if they necessitate that I grow and change." You want your sleep thinking prompt to operate at that level of depth and honesty. Double-check to make sure that your sleep thinking prompt is brimming over with authenticity.

Journal Prompt: "I may not be comfortable with change, but I understand why it may sometimes—even often— be necessary."

_____

_____

_____

_____

Sleep Thinking Prompt: "I wonder what it would feel like to make the changes I need to make."

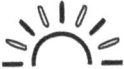

_____

_____

_____

_____

Morning Processing:

_____

_____

_____

_____

_____

_____

_____

_____

30

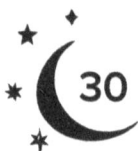

BEGIN IN WONDER

"Wisdom begins in wonder."
—SOCRATES

Your sleep thinking prompt invites you to wonder, not to "think hard," worry, investigate, or anything else. Do you remember, as a child, having a wonder like, "I wonder why the sky is blue"? You weren't worried about the sky being blue. You weren't really demanding a scientific answer. You were imagining, speculating, wondering, wandering, dreaming. Your sleep thinking prompt is like that: a portal to deep speculation. If you can imbue your sleep thinking prompt with a sense of wonder, your results will amaze you.

Journal Prompt: "I think I understand what it means to 'wonder.' I think it means the following"

_____

_____

_____

_____

Sleep Thinking Prompt: "I wonder what I might learn if I wondered more."

_____

_____

_____

_____

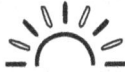

Morning Processing:

_____

_____

_____

_____

_____

_____

_____

_____

_____

31

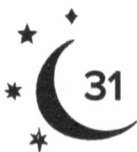

I'LL TAKE CARE OF THAT

"If a writer is hesitant to go deeply into a character, the brain says, 'Okay, you go to sleep, I'll take care of it. I'll show you where that is.'"
—MAYA ANGELOU

You've changed your bedtime routine to support your sleep thinking. You've readied yourself for bed. You've thought or said your sleep thinking prompt. Is there anything left to do? Yes, sleep. You want all this leading up to sleep to lead to sleep. You want to go to sleep and sleep like a baby. This means relaxing, surrendering, and disappearing into the night. Let yourself float off, without a thought or a worry in the world.

Journal Prompt: "I think I may still be a little hesitant to float off to sleep. I think that might be the case for the following reasons."

_____

_____

_____

Sleep Thinking Prompt: "I wonder what it would be like to just drift off to sleep."

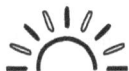

_____

_____

_____

Morning Processing:

_____

_____

_____

_____

_____

_____

_____

_____

_____

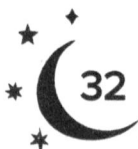

WHEN THINGS COME ALIVE

"Night, when words fade and things come alive."
—ANTOINE ST. EXUPÉRY

Your sleep may prove turbulent. This may be true whether or not you are making use of your sleep thinking, whether or not some particular thing is bothering you, whether or not anything special is going on in your life. Your sleep may prove turbulent just because you are full of an aliveness that is playing itself out while you sleep. You may be tossing and turning not because you are worrying, but because you are on some quest, some amazing adventure. Don't suppose that all sleep turbulence is the sign of a problem."

Journal Prompt: "I think that for the following reasons I will worry less about the turbulence of my sleep."

_____

_____

_____

_____

Sleep Thinking Prompt: "I wonder what adventure I'll be going on tonight."

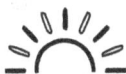

_____

_____

_____

_____

Morning Processing:

_____

_____

_____

_____

_____

_____

_____

_____

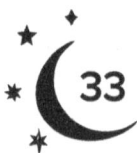

33

THE PACT

"There is between sleep and us something like a pact;
it is agreed that sleep will become domesticated
and serve as an instrument of our power."
—MAURICE BLANCHOT

Well, maybe not domesticated. But there is indeed a pact to be made between us and sleep. We agree to serve one another. We will go to bed properly, surrender to sleep, treat it with respect, and honor its value. It, in turn, will restore us, provide us with nightly adventures, and sleep-think solutions to our problems. This is a pact made not between lord and servant, but between partners.

Journal Prompt: "I would like to craft the following pact with sleep."

_____

_____

_____

_____

Sleep Thinking Prompt: "I wonder what it would be like to partner with sleep."

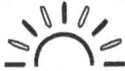

_____

_____

_____

_____

Morning Processing:

_____

_____

_____

_____

_____

_____

_____

_____

34

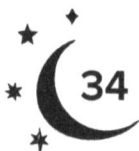

THE RIGHT QUESTION

"In the morning I wake up and think,
okay, where am I? What's going on?
Do I have any ideas? And usually I do."
—ELMORE LEONARD

When you wake up, the right question isn't "What should I have for breakfast?" or "What ordeals am I facing today?" The right question is some version of "What would my sleep thinking like to provide me with this morning?" Your best bet is to turn to your sleep thinking, not to the new day. You might use Elmore Leonard's prompt, "Do I have any ideas?" Or you might repeat your sleep thinking prompt of the previous night and see what wants to percolate up. The main thing is that you honor your intention that, first thing each morning, you process the night.

Journal Prompt: "How can I aim myself in the direction of processing the night if, when I wake up, my mind wants to turn to the new day?"

_____

_____

_____

_____

Sleep Thinking Prompt: "I wonder what my best wake-up routine might be."

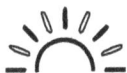

_____

_____

_____

_____

Morning Processing:

_____

_____

_____

_____

_____

_____

_____

_____

35

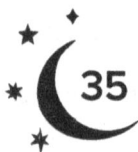

MORNING IS BEST

"Morning is the best and most suitable time for work, because we are then rejuvenated, flexible and energetic."
—GEORG ALFRED TIENES

If you're intending to make use of your sleep thinking, you need to turn to it first thing when you awake. I am calling the time when you awake "morning" because most people sleep at night and wake up in the morning. But more than ten million adults work shifts that have them working at night and sleeping during the day. However, the same idea holds for them: they would want to turn to their sleep thinking as soon as they awake, even if that is four in the afternoon. The main point is that you will want to turn to your sleep thinking first thing, or else it will evaporate as your mind contemplates the realities of a new day.

Journal Prompt: "I think I can get to my sleep thinking first thing when I awake if I carefully create a plan and follow it."

_____

_____

_____

_____

Sleep Thinking Prompt: "I wonder what my brain will want to offer me as soon as I awaken."

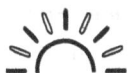

_____

_____

_____

_____

Morning Processing:

_____

_____

_____

_____

_____

36

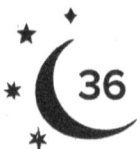

HELLO, SOLUTION

"I woke up with the solution."
—THOMAS EDISON

Be ready for the solutions that are coming. That they have come is no more surprising than that the sun has risen. Your full brain worked on the problem, gave it a lot of thought, and arrived at a conclusion. Of course, this is not a result to expect every single morning. Some mathematical problems have not been solved in the centuries since they were posed! That would be a lot of waiting, if one waited every day for a solution to that sort of puzzle. But for many of our problems, issues, and challenges, answers are just around the corner. And when a solution comes, smile. You just used your brain brilliantly!

Journal Prompt: "When a solution comes, I will celebrate in the following ways."

_____

_____

_____

Sleep Thinking Prompt: "I wonder if tonight is the night that an answer arrives."

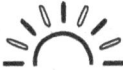

_____

_____

_____

Morning Processing:

_____

_____

_____

_____

_____

_____

_____

_____

_____

_____

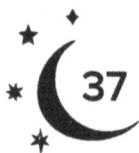

INTERPRETATIONS

"A transformative dream carries with it sufficient
meaning to tell the dreamer what he needs to know."
—LEE WOLDENBERG

Historically, dreams have been thought to need interpreting. What did that cigar mean? What did that unicorn mean? What did it mean that that my friends had no faces? The information you receive from sleep thinking likely also needs interpreting. Maybe it has become clear to you, via your sleep thinking, that the main character in your novel should be Portuguese and not Spanish. But why? What does that really mean? And what does it imply for the novel's structure and arc? That you now "know" that your main character will be Portuguese isn't a final destination. A lot more considering is required!

Journal Prompt: "When I receive information from my sleep thinking, I'll interpret that information using the following tactics and strategies."

_____

_____

Sleep Thinking Prompt: "I wonder if tonight's sleep thinking solution might come already interpreted."

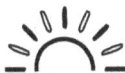

_____

_____

_____

_____

Morning Processing:

_____

_____

_____

_____

_____

_____

_____

_____

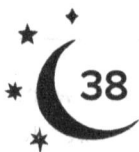

CONNECTING THE DOTS

"Information is not knowledge."
—ALBERT EINSTEIN

We want to know, not just acquire information. Let's say that you're about to purchase a home. You're torn between two homes, and your sleep thinking provides you with bits of information that you hadn't noticed while awake: that one home is near railroad tracks and that the other is near power lines. No doubt, that is very useful information. But that isn't an answer! And even if your sleeping thinking seemed to point in one direction or the other, could you simply trust it, or would you still have to think some more? You know the answer to that one. More thinking required!

Journal Prompt: "In the following ways, I will honor my commitment to continue the thinking that my sleep thinking has begun."

_____

_____

_____

Sleep Thinking Prompt: "I wonder if I might be provided with some knowledge tonight, and not just information."

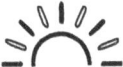

_____

_____

_____

Morning Processing:

_____

_____

_____

_____

_____

_____

_____

_____

_____

39

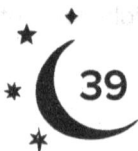

APPLYING KNOWLEDGE

*"Knowledge is of no value unless
you put it into practice."*
—ANTON CHEKHOV

You move from information to knowledge. Then you move on to action. Probably, you will experience both resistance and anxiety as you contemplate this next important step. You may have learned that you must spend money on something you hoped would be free, that you must move painfully slowly, step by step, to reach your goal, that you must have a hard conversation with a loved one, and so on. How will you tackle this natural resistance and manage this natural anxiety?

Journal Prompt: "I intend to handle the resistance and anxiety that may follow my sleep thinking efforts by committing to the following program."

_____

_____

_____

Sleep Thinking Prompt: "I wonder what might be the best way to handle any resistance or anxiety that pops up during this process."

_____

_____

_____

Morning Processing:

_____

_____

_____

_____

_____

_____

_____

_____

_____

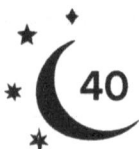

PRACTICALITIES

*"I am a practical dreamer. My
dreams are not airy things."*
—MOHANDAS GANDHI

Our sleep thinking provides us with a lot: solutions, ideas, next steps, visions. Then we are obliged to employ our waking mind to make use of what we have been given.

That we now have a picture of a solution is not the same as having solved the problem in real life. Maybe our sleep thinking has made it clear that we can't handle our addiction without twelve-step support. Then it is on us to find a meeting and go to a meeting. Not following up robs sleep thinking of its power and value.

Journal Prompt: "I know it may prove hard to move from insight to action, but I intend to help myself do exactly that by doing the following."

_____

_____

_____

Sleep Thinking Prompt: "I wonder how I'm going to turn the answers I'm getting into the reality of action."

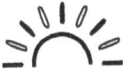

_____

_____

_____

Morning Processing:

_____

_____

_____

_____

_____

_____

_____

_____

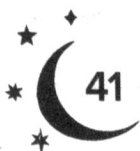

OBEY THE NIGHT

"It is wise to obey the night."
—HOMER

An answer is often—even usually—just the beginning. What typically follows is the heavy lifting of real work to do. If you received an excellent solution to your problem—say, the design for the business you've been percolating—well, now comes actually building the business. That reality, that work necessarily follows insight, can make you wonder whether you even want to sleep think. Let's recommit to sleep thinking right now. The power of sleep thinking is incredibly valuable to you, even if it makes work.

Journal Prompt: "I understand that I might want to table my brain's own power, so as to avoid hard truths and hard work, but I'll keep myself from doing that in the following ways."

_____

_____

_____

Sleep Thinking Prompt: "I wonder how I can keep myself committed to sleep thinking."

_____

_____

_____

Morning Processing:

_____

_____

_____

_____

_____

_____

_____

_____

_____

42

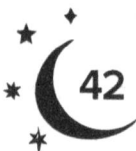

NOT SWIFT, NOT EASY

"I was taught that the way of progress
was neither swift nor easy."
—MARIE CURIE

The progress you may make writing your novel, building your business, losing weight, reducing the stresses in your life, or improving your relationship with your mate may feel painfully slow—and so subtle that you aren't sure that you are even making progress. So it is easy not to want to keep track of your progress, out of fear that there isn't much to record. But keeping track is a good idea and part of the process. How will you do that?

Journal Prompt: "I intend to keep track of my progress in the following ways."

_____

_____

_____

_____

Sleep Thinking Prompt: "I wonder if I might get a little confirmation of my progress tonight."

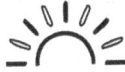

_____

_____

_____

_____

Morning Processing:

_____

_____

_____

_____

_____

_____

_____

_____

_____

43

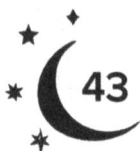

THE CONVICTION TO REPEAT

"Constant repetition carries conviction."
—ROBERT COLLIER

Maybe you've had good luck using sleep thinking to solve a tricky problem. Congratulations! But is that somehow a reason not to continue the sleep thinking process? Not at all. Keep the habit of sleep thinking alive by identifying other, maybe half-buried, issues, concerns, or problems to ponder. Sleep think your new suite of paintings, revisit your desire to move abroad, reevaluate your decision not to foster children. Isn't there always something to wonder about?

Journal Prompt: "Once I'm finished sleep thinking one challenge, problem, or issue, I'll move right on to sleep thinking the next according to the following procedure."

_____

_____

_____

_____

Sleep Thinking Prompt: "I wonder what will happen offering up this new problem to my sleeping brain."

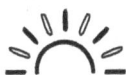

_____

_____

_____

_____

Morning Processing:

_____

_____

_____

_____

_____

_____

_____

_____

_____

44

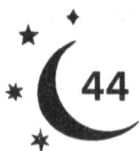

THE LOOM OF LIFE NEVER STOPS

*"We sleep, but the loom of life never stops, and the
pattern which was weaving when the sun went down
is weaving when it comes up in the morning."*
—HENRY WARD BEECHER

Consider bringing the fundamentals of sleep thinking to your daytime thinking. What might that look like? Well, that would mean that you had committed to silence; that you posed yourself a wonder, rather than a hard-edged demand or an anxious worry; that you surrendered your grip on your mind and invited your brain to "do its thing"; that you calmly and quietly waited; that you stood open and ready to receive what your brain had to offer; and that you took that new information and moved on to turning it into knowledge and action. Maybe you'd like to try that today or tomorrow?

Journal Prompt: "I can imagine using the fundamentals of sleep thinking during my waking hours in the following ways."

_____

_____

_____

_____

Sleep Thinking Prompt: "I wonder how I might apply sleep thinking during the day."

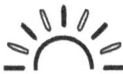

_____

_____

_____

_____

Morning Processing:

_____

_____

_____

_____

_____

_____

_____

_____

45

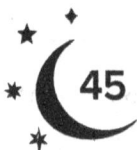

LONGING FOR WAYS

"It's amazing how the unconscious longs
for ways to get in touch with us."
—SUE GRAFTON

We haven't used the word "unconscious" so far in our discussions. Is sleep thinking a form of "accessing the unconscious?" Well, that would depend a lot on what that construct means and represents. Is it a place full of what Jung called archetypes, as if it were a busy bus station? Is it a place roiling with shameful fantasies, repressed desires, tyrannical rules, and other powerful id material, as Freud supposed? Or is it simply that which is going on just outside of conscious awareness, something happening in the next room behind a closed and locked door? And, as Sue Grafton puts it, is it something longing for ways to be in touch?

Journal Prompt: "I think I would describe my unconscious in the following ways."

_____

_____

_____

_____

Sleep Thinking Prompt: "I wonder what my unconscious would like to provide me with tonight."

_____

_____

_____

_____

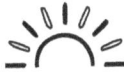

Morning Processing:

_____

_____

_____

_____

_____

_____

_____

_____

46

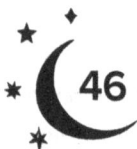

WHAT TEMPTATION RESISTED?

"We should every night call ourselves to an account. What infirmity have I mastered today? What passions opposed? What temptation resisted? What virtue acquired?"
—SENECA

You might usefully employ sleep thinking as part of your addiction recovery program, if you are working such a program. You might try as a sleep thinking prompt, "I wonder how I should handle that triggering event that's coming up on Thursday," or "I wonder why I'm having such trouble making amends." If you're not in a recovery program but suspect that you ought to be, your prompt might be something like, "I wonder if it's time to take the downside of my drinking seriously."

Journal Prompt: "How might I use sleep thinking as part of my recovery program?"

_____

_____

_____

_____

Sleep Thinking Prompt: "I wonder if my sleeping brain might like to help me with my recovery."

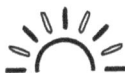

_____

_____

_____

_____

Morning Processing:

_____

_____

_____

_____

_____

_____

_____

47

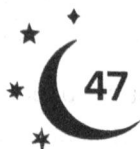

WHO YOU ARE IN THE DARK

"All great revolutions occur at night!
Character is who you are in the dark."
—BUCKAROO BANZAI

Is there some aspect of your personality that you'd like to upgrade? Maybe you'd like to become less caustic and critical, or more passionate and spontaneous, or calmer and more centered? Let your sleeping brain help! Invite personality upgrades while you sleep. You might try a sleep thinking prompt of the following sort: "I wonder what's the best way to become the person I would really love to be."

Journal Prompt: "How might I use sleep thinking to upgrade my personality?"

_____

_____

_____

_____

Sleep Thinking Prompt: "I wonder what in my personality or character is holding me back."

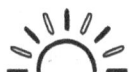

Morning Processing:

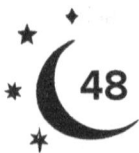

48

RECENCY

"Reports from deep sleep make the most sense to subjects in terms of references to recent experiences in their life."
—DAVID FOULKES

Maybe something very important happened recently, even as recently as today, but you're too preoccupied and too busy to take any real notice of it. Let your sleep thinking help you. You might try as a sleep thinking prompt something like, "I wonder why that conversation with Harriet is still bothering me," or "I wonder why that bit of world news struck me as so troubling." When you have the intuition that something important happened, try not to let the event, and the information it may be carrying, slip on by.

Journal Prompt: "I think I might use my sleep thinking in the following ways to keep track of important events as they occur."

_____

_____

_____

_____

Sleep Thinking Prompt: "I wonder why what happened today is bothering me so much."

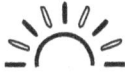

_____

_____

_____

_____

Morning Processing:

_____

_____

_____

_____

_____

_____

_____

_____

49

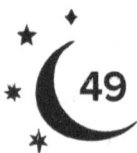

THE BEST MEDITATION

"Sleep is the best meditation."
—THE DALAI LAMA

Perhaps you're already a practiced meditator. Or maybe you have no experience with meditation. In either case, you can make use of your sleep thinking in exactly the same ways that meditating supports mindfulness. For instance, you might invite your sleeping brain not to think, but rather to let thoughts pass on through without remarking on them, worrying about them, or being stung by them. How might your brain react to such a prompt? Aren't you a little bit curious?

Journal Prompt: "I think I can see the following connections between sleep thinking and meditation."

_____

_____

_____

_____

Sleep Thinking Prompt: "I wonder what it would be like to not attach to my thoughts."

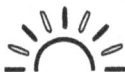

_____

_____

_____

_____

Morning Processing:

_____

_____

_____

_____

_____

_____

_____

_____

50

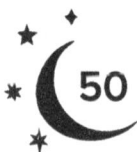

OUR ACCESS TO OTHER WORLDS

"I've always had access to other worlds.
We all do, because we all dream."
—LEONORA CARRINGTON

Surrealism. The Multiverse. Mystery. Other worlds. Most of the day, we are rather solidly rooted in this reality and can't help but pay attention to catching the bus, picking up groceries, getting some more work done, and all the rest. But part of us desperately wishes that we could wander off somewhere far away, somewhere further than a sixteen-hour flight can take us. Use your sleep thinking to travel as far as you like.

Journal Prompt: "I can see the following connections between surrealism and sleep thinking."

_____

_____

_____

_____

Sleep Thinking Prompt: "I wonder where my night brain would like to take me tonight."

_____

_____

_____

_____

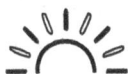

Morning Processing:

_____

_____

_____

_____

_____

_____

_____

_____

_____

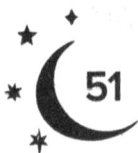

51

POEMS FULLY WRITTEN

"In sleep, human beings are brought back to themselves, having sloughed off everything else. Some have returned with poems fully written or equations solved."
—GABRIELLE ROY

There is absolutely nothing better for your creative life than employing sleep thinking. Harnessing your brain's natural power to think while the body sleeps can make the difference between creating deeply and not creating at all. That is not hyperbole. If you are not employing your sleep thinking, you may well not be connected to your creativity at all. Because, if you were connected, wouldn't your brain want to continue its fascinating pursuits at every opportunity? Given that it can sleep think—why would it not want to?

Journal Prompt: "For the following reasons, I recognize that sleep thinking may be profoundly important for my creative life."

_____

_____

_____

_____

Sleep Thinking Prompt: "I wonder into what creative project I'd really like to throw myself."

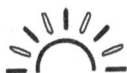

_____

_____

_____

_____

Morning Processing:

_____

_____

_____

_____

_____

_____

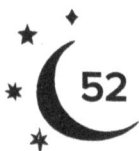

THE TOUGHEST PROBLEMS

"It's a common experience that a problem difficult at night is resolved in the morning after the committee of sleep has worked on it."
—JOHN STEINBECK

You've just received a cancer diagnosis. How will you tell the children? Your elderly mother is losing her memory. How will you take care of her? Your business is facing financial ruin. Is there any way to save it? A dictator has taken over your country. How are you supposed to react to that? Can sleep thinking help with problems that are this awful? Yes. Your sleep thinking will provide you with options, possibilities, maybe even answers, and rays of hope.

Journal Prompt: "I will employ my sleep thinking power in the following ways when the problem seems awful to face or impossible to solve."

_____

_____

_____

Sleep Thinking Prompt: "I wonder how I should deal with this terrible thing I'm facing."

_____

_____

_____

Morning Processing:

_____

_____

_____

_____

_____

_____

_____

_____

_____

_____

53

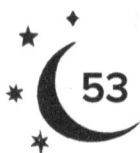

WHAT WE WISH FOR WAKING

"We see sleeping what we wish for waking."
—GEORGE PETTIE

What are you wishing for? Invite your brain to help by having it envision your wishes fulfilled. Invite it to spend a portion of the night throwing you a party in honor of winning that award you covet so much. Invite it to spend an hour tooling about the lake in the boat you dream of owning. Seeing success helps keep you motivated on the path to success. Use your sleep thinking to support your dreams and desires.

Journal Prompt: "I can see using sleep thinking to support my dreams, desires, and goals in the following ways."

_____

_____

_____

_____

_____

Sleep Thinking Prompt: "I wonder what it would look like to have my wish fulfilled."

_____

_____

_____

_____

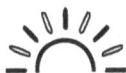

Morning Processing:

_____

_____

_____

_____

_____

_____

_____

_____

_____

54

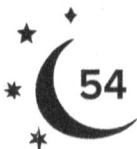

AT EASE WITH NOT YET KNOWING

"Being at ease with not knowing is crucial
for answers to come to you."
—ECKHART TOLLE

You're a chemist, and you've been working at picturing the structure of a certain molecule. You've invited your brain to work on it during sleep, and this morning you receive the information that the answer has something to do with coiled snakes. But you can't make sense of the information. What should you do? Throw up your hands? No. Your best response is to be easy. Be easy with not yet knowing what "coiled snakes" means. The answer is likely coming. Be easy with not yet knowing!

Journal Prompt: "If I can't interpret the information that my sleep thinking has provided me with yet, I'll react in the following ways."

_____

_____

_____

Sleep Thinking Prompt: "I wonder what the full answer might be."

_____

_____

_____

Morning Processing:

_____

_____

_____

_____

_____

_____

_____

_____

_____

_____

55

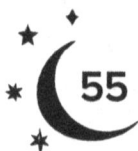

HOW LONG SHOULD IT TAKE?

"Waiting is painful."
—PAULO COELHO

You wake up and sit ready to process the night. Nothing. The next morning, nothing. You change your sleep thinking prompt. Again, nothing. You reexamine the problem to see if the way you're framing it needs tweaking. You tweak it. You create a new sleep thinking prompt. Nothing. You give up for a day. Of course, nothing. You try a different bedtime routine. Nothing. The problem hasn't eased; a solution is still wanted. How long should this take? Well, you know the answer. As long as it takes.

Journal Prompt: "I'll use the following strategies to not give up on sleep thinking when the sleep thinking process is taking a long time, or if it seems not to be working."

_____

_____

_____

Sleep Thinking Prompt: "I wonder if an answer would like to come tomorrow."

_____

_____

_____

Morning Processing:

_____

_____

_____

_____

_____

_____

_____

_____

_____

56

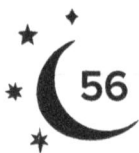

DECISION IS A RISK

"Decision is a risk rooted in the courage of being free."
—PAUL TILLICH

How can you know if you've chosen the right sleep thinking prompt? Well, first, you might check to see if it perhaps feels slightly off. If it does, tweak it and play with it until it feels as right as, in that moment, it can. Then you will simply have to give it a try. Maybe it is exactly right; maybe it isn't. You can only tell by trying—and even then, unless the answer comes to you first thing the next morning, you may still not be sure. Did the answer not come because you got the prompt wrong, or because the answer isn't available yet? These are the questions that freedom poses.

Journal Prompt: "I think I can learn over time how to create sleep thinking prompts that work. I can do this by employing the following plan."

_____

_____

_____

Sleep Thinking Prompt: "I wonder, brain, if you'd like to tackle a sleep thinking prompt different from the one we've been trying."

_____

_____

_____

Morning Processing:

_____

_____

_____

_____

_____

_____

_____

_____

_____

_____

57

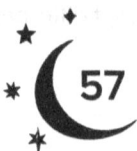

BY SEEKING AND BLUNDERING

"By seeking and blundering, we learn."
—JOHANN WOLFGANG VON GOETHE

You are working on a novel. You aren't sure whether to set the second half in Barcelona or Seville. You sleep think on it and get clear reasons for setting it in Seville. So you do. Ten thousand words later, you realize that it really has to be Barcelona. Did you blunder? Yes and no. Your brain gave you the best answer it could at that moment. But it couldn't give you a guarantee. That will always be the case with sleep thinking. You will get wonderful answers very often—but not always. How could it be always?

Journal Prompt: "For the following reasons, I am easy in the knowledge that sleep thinking answers do not come with guarantees as to their ultimate correctness."

_____

_____

_____

Sleep Thinking Prompt: "Brain, I wonder what you would like to provide me with tonight."

_____

_____

_____

Morning Processing:

_____

_____

_____

_____

_____

_____

_____

_____

_____

_____

_____

58

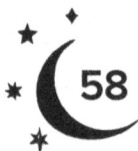

A FORM OF NOT BEING SURE

"Living is a form of not being sure."
—AGNES DE MILLE

Needing certainty is a trap. Life is a series of experiments whose outcomes can't be known in advance. You'll want to treat your sleep thinking results in that context. Maybe you have something important that you need to say to your daughter. Your sleep thinking provides you with something you might say. You nod: What you've been provided with sounds good. But will your daughter react exactly as you hope she'll react? Who can say? Of course, you're not sure. That's life: a form of not being sure.

Journal Prompt: "I have the following plan for dealing with the reality that our life choices come with inevitable uncertainties."

_____

_____

_____

Sleep Thinking Prompt: "I wonder how best to live without assurances."

_____

_____

_____

☼ Morning Processing:

_____

_____

_____

_____

_____

_____

_____

_____

_____

_____

59

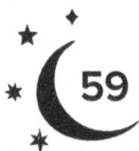

FROM PROBLEM TO QUESTION

"When you encounter a problem you cannot solve, turn it into a question you can explore."
—PETER BLOCK

You identify a problem, create a sleep thinking prompt, and invite your brain to think as you sleep. That is one sense of moving from problem to question. There is a second sense, too. Your sleep thinking may provide you with lots of good information, but not with a complete answer. So, now you have a new problem, making sense of that information. You could stew about this; or you could turn the matter over to your brain with a new sleep thinking question. This is our rhythm: Problem begets question; question begets useful information but not a complete solution; this creates a new problem...which begets a new question!

Journal Prompt: "I would describe this rhythm of problem leading to question leading to new problem leading to new question in the following way."

_____

_____

_____

_____

Sleep Thinking Prompt: "Okay, brain, here is my new
question, flowing from what you gave me last night."

_____

_____

_____

_____

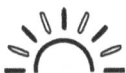

Morning Processing:

_____

_____

_____

_____

_____

_____

_____

60

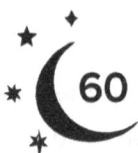

WHEN THE ANSWER IS MATURITY

"Sometimes problems don't require a solution to solve them; instead they require maturity to outgrow them."
— STEVE MARABOLI

Some problems can't be solved because we haven't grown into the person who could solve them. We may have to wait—even a long time. Imagine trying to solve a vexing relationship issue with your mate while the two of you are drinking alcoholically. Isn't sobriety the real agenda issue? Increased self-awareness and a leap in maturity may be needed before a problem can be solved. Might that be something valuable to sleep think about?

Journal Prompt: "Let me have a frank discussion with myself about my readiness to solve the problems facing me."

_____

_____

_____

_____

Sleep Thinking Prompt: "I wonder if I should focus on growth, maturity, and personal responsibility?"

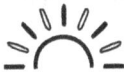

_____

_____

_____

_____

Morning Processing:

_____

_____

_____

_____

_____

_____

_____

_____

_____

61

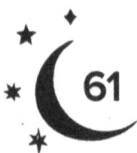

PARALYSIS BY ANALYSIS

"Too much thinking leads to paralysis by analysis."
—ROBERT HERJAVEC

No doubt there are certain dangers associated with inviting your brain to do its best thinking. One danger might be that you make discoveries that disturb you, confound you, or provoke you. You may not like the solutions your brain provides, ever though they are the best ones. Or maybe you mistakenly conclude that your work is done, just because you can picture the solution. But that you have arrived at a solution is not the same thing as having implemented that solution!

Journal Prompt: "I think that sleep thinking might sometimes feel 'dangerous' for the following reasons."

_____

_____

_____

_____

Sleep Thinking Prompt: "I wonder if my sleep thinking always has to feel safe."

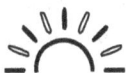

_____

_____

_____

_____

Morning Processing:

_____

_____

_____

_____

_____

_____

_____

_____

62

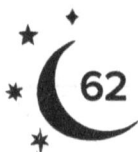

THE SONG WON'T LET YOU

"You try to sleep, but the song won't let you. So you have to get up and make it into something and then you're allowed to sleep."
—JOHN LENNON

Folks sometimes worry that inviting their brain to think will cause them to have ideas in the middle of the night that, by their vivacity and pressing nature, force them to wake up. That may happen, though only rarely. But even if it were to happen, all that would mean is that your brain had just provided you with a good idea! Write it down and get back to sleep, or stay awake for a bit and enjoy elaborating on that idea. If a good idea wakes you up, that isn't a tragedy. Of course, you wouldn't want this to happen every night, to the point of insomnia. But if happens only occasionally, that is no particular problem.

Journal Prompt: "Am I certain that I'm okay with ideas waking me up occasionally?"

_____

_____

_____

_____

Sleep Thinking Prompt: "I wonder what it would be like if a great idea woke me up in the middle of the night tonight!"

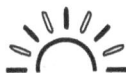

_____

_____

_____

_____

Morning Processing:

_____

_____

_____

_____

_____

_____

_____

63

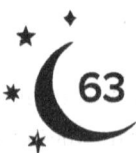

DARE TO VISUALIZE

"Dare to visualize a world in which your most treasured dreams have become true."
— RALPH MARSTON

A guided visualization is a scenario you create for yourself to help you picture something you want to have happen. Maybe the scenario has to do with your healthy cells defeating your cancer cells, with you achieving calmness as you walk through the woods on the way to a lake, or with you performing the songs you've written before a packed audience of thousands. You can create guided visualizations when you're awake; and you can also invite your brain to create them while you sleep. Wouldn't that put a smile on your face, to wake up to the memory of something visualized and realized?

Journal Prompt: "I think I would like to invite my brain to create the following guided visualizations."

_____

_____

Sleep Thinking Prompt: "Brain, I wonder if you might provide me with a full-length movie of me succeeding."

_____

_____

_____

_____

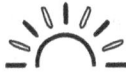

Morning Processing:

_____

_____

_____

_____

_____

_____

_____

_____

64

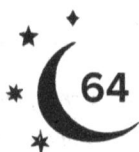

TO UNDERSTAND THE
IMMEASURABLE

"To understand the immeasurable, the mind must be extraordinarily quiet, still."
– J. Krishnamurti

A meditation is a spoken or written reflective piece that explores a particular idea, experience, or question with depth and intention. The questions explored might be philosophical, spiritual, or personal in nature. For example, Marcus Aurelius' *Meditations* are philosophical reflections on Stoic principles. Might you like to invite your brain to create a meditation while you sleep? Wouldn't it be a good idea to explore your biggest questions, about the universe and life itself, when everything is at its stillest?

Journal Prompt: "For the following reasons, I think it might prove valuable to sleep think meditations into existence."

_____

_____

_____

Sleep thinking Prompt: "I wonder what it would be like to receive a meditation tonight."

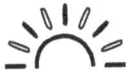

_____

_____

_____

_____

Morning Processing:

_____

_____

_____

_____

_____

_____

_____

_____

_____

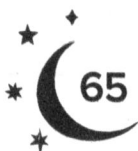

65

A BIG SHADOW

"Worry often gives a small thing a big shadow."
—SWEDISH PROVERB

I've been inviting you to go to sleep with a wonder rather than a worry. But worries aren't that easy to dismiss. They have the power to linger, to force themselves upon us, to rob us of the work of neurons that might otherwise be much better employed. So, that might mean adding an anxiety management tactic to your bedtime routine. Maybe a soothing meditation? Maybe a small calming ceremony? Maybe a relaxing guided visualization? What might you include so that you move from worry to wonder as you get ready for bed?

Journal Prompt: "I will use the following methods to move from worry to wonder as I prepare for bed."

_____

_____

_____

Sleep Thinking Prompt: "I wonder what's the best way to release worry."

_____

_____

_____

Morning Processing:

_____

_____

_____

_____

_____

_____

_____

_____

_____

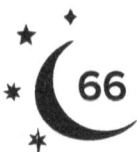

66

ON NAPPING

*"Never go to sleep without a request
to your subconscious."*
—THOMAS EDISON

So far, we've focused on your night sleep thinking. But your brain also thinks while you nap. Naps, like all sleep, are wonderful for gathering your thoughts, working out problems, connecting the dots, and allowing your imagination free play. As with night sleep thinking, a good policy is to start your nap with, as Edison puts it, "a request to your subconscious"—what I've been calling a sleep thinking prompt. Then, on to your nap—and to the answers that await you!

Journal Prompt: "I can see the following advantages to using napping to sleep think."

_____

_____

_____

Sleep Thinking Prompt: "Let me nap think that solution!"

_____

_____

_____

Morning Processing:

_____

_____

_____

_____

_____

_____

_____

_____

_____

_____

67

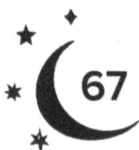

A MENTAL SIMMER

"My stories run up and bite me on the leg—
I respond by writing them down—everything goes
onto a kind of mental simmer while I sleep."
—RAY BRADBURY

Life comes down to making one choice after another. This is certainly true of the creative process, which is exactly about choosing. What choices might a creative face? Whether to write a memoir or, to play it safer, a novel. Whether to opt for composing a string quartet or a symphony. Where to put a dab of color, what word comes next, what note comes next. All that choosing, all that simmering! Wouldn't it be lovely to quiet that tumult by sleeping—and letting your brain work at its best in silence?

Journal Prompt: "I think I see the following connections between sleep thinking and effortless choosing."

_____

_____

_____

Sleep Thinking Prompt: "Brain, here is the stew I've been simmering! What might you make of it?"

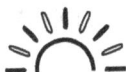

_____

_____

_____

Morning Processing:

_____

_____

_____

_____

_____

_____

_____

_____

_____

68

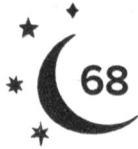

ON NOT WAITING FOR
THE RIGHT MOOD

"I don't wait for moods. You accomplish
nothing if you do that. Your mind must
know it has got to get down to work."
—PEARL S. BUCK

Pearl Buck's advice applies to both day thinking and night thinking. Often, we aren't in the mood to think (or to do much of anything). Or maybe we've adopted the notion that we can't create or think until we get "in the right mood." It would be good to unlearn these ideas and to announce that you have thinking to do, so as to solve your problems, reduce your stress, and get on with your creative work, irrespective of what mood you're in. This is the message to share with your brain: "Forget about mood! Let's get on with living and thinking."

Journal Prompt: "I will deal with my moods in the following ways."

_____

_____

_____

_____

Sleep Thinking Prompt: "I wonder what it would be like to always be in the mood to think."

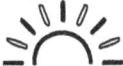

_____

_____

_____

_____

Morning Processing:

_____

_____

_____

_____

_____

69

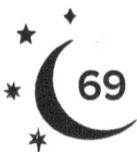

ON NOT WAITING ON THE MUSE

"Show up, show up, show up, and after
a while the muse shows up, too."
—ISABEL ALLENDE

Maybe you're a creative person who's gotten into the habit of waiting on the muse. You may believe that it's better to wait for inspiration than to sit down and see what wants to percolate up. In my experience, a lot of time gets wasted that way—and inspiration may have a way of never arriving. Instead, turn your sleep thinking into a robust practice, where every night you go to bed with a wonder and every morning you turn directly to your work, rightly presuming that something excellent will be there. Doesn't that sound better than waiting?

Journal Prompt: "I think the following are good reasons for not waiting for inspiration."

_____

_____

_____

Sleep Thinking Prompt: "I wonder what lyrics might perfectly complete that song I'm working on."

_____

_____

_____

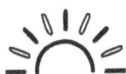

Morning Processing:

_____

_____

_____

_____

_____

_____

_____

_____

_____

70

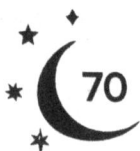

YOU WILL NEVER LIVE

*"You will never live if you are looking
for the meaning of life."*
—ALBERT CAMUS

My belief is that meaning is not something to seek, because it isn't "out there" anywhere. Rather, it is a special sort of psychological experience, one that we can coax into being by learning how to "make meaning." Just as we can become happier by learning what actually makes us happy, we can live a more meaningful life by identifying what actually stirs up that special feeling of meaning in us. Might this be something to sleep think about? Indeed, is anything more important to ponder?

Journal Prompt: "I see the following differences between the idea of 'seeking meaning' and the idea of 'making meaning.' "

_____

_____

_____

Sleep Thinking Prompt: "I wonder, what in life have I experienced as truly meaningful?"

_____

_____

_____

Morning Processing:

_____

_____

_____

_____

_____

_____

_____

_____

_____

71

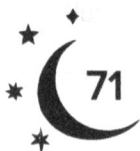

THE PRIVILEGE OF A LIFETIME

"The privilege of a lifetime is to become who you truly are."
—CARL JUNG

I've described how sleep thinking can help you solve your problems, connect to your creative work, reduce your stress, and more. But what it can also do is help you become the person you want to become, the person you have always been meant to be. It can help you create your life in your own image. By inviting your brain to dive deeply into the contours of your original personality, to read and respond to the blueprint of who you were meant to be, you can grow into your authentic self as you sleep. That, as Jung puts it, is the "privilege of a lifetime."

Journal Prompt: "I see that I can use sleep thinking in the following ways to become the person I really want to be."

Sleep Thinking Prompt: "I wonder, brain, what picture do you see of the me that I might want to be?"

_____

_____

_____

Morning Processing:

_____

_____

_____

_____

_____

_____

_____

_____

_____

_____

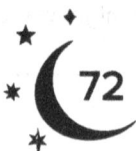

72

HAVING A WHY

"He who has a why to live can bear almost any how."
—FRIEDRICH NIETZSCHE

We are entitled to multiple life purposes. Many things are important to us; we have many whys to live. But most people haven't entertained the thought that they have multiple life purposes available to them. So they keep seeking purpose and pining for purpose. Try sleep thinking on the proposition, "I wonder what my many life purposes might be." You might learn something really astounding!

Journal Prompt: "What are my thoughts about the differences between 'the purpose of life' and the idea of multiple life purposes?"

_____

_____

_____

_____

Sleep Thinking Prompt: "I wonder, which of my many life purposes should I focus on tonight?"

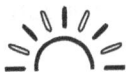

_____

_____

_____

_____

Morning Processing:

_____

_____

_____

_____

_____

_____

_____

_____

73

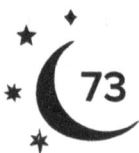

A HOPE THAT'S WAITING

"There's a hope that's waiting for you in the dark."
—CARL JUNG

The very idea of sleep thinking should make you a little hopeful, cheerful, and optimistic. That your brain can do such excellent work while you sleep, and then deliver up its results the very next morning, is something to smile about. If all we had were our waking thoughts, all those fragments, all that noise, all that self-pestering, our brain wouldn't seem like that much of a prize. But add in sleep thinking, and that gives us a very different picture of our brain. Our brain is rather better at what it does than we thought it was! A little applause, please.

Journal Prompt: "In the following ways, learning about sleep thinking has made me positively reappraise how I view my brain."

_____

_____

_____

Sleep Thinking Prompt: "I wonder what else my brain can do!"

_____

_____

_____

Morning Processing:

_____

_____

_____

_____

_____

_____

_____

_____

_____

_____

74

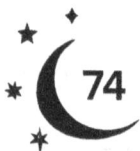

THE NOON OF THOUGHT

"The dead of midnight is the noon of thought."
—ANNA LETITIA BARBAULD

I hope that you will not only use sleep thinking—to solve your problems, to reduce your stress, to increase your creativity—but that you will fall in love with this special human resource. There is nothing quite like it. You might even announce that, as one of your life purposes, as one of those things that's most important to you, you will explore your natural ability to sleep think in a systematic way, but making it an every-night practice. You'll find it endlessly useful—and simply brilliant!

Journal Prompt: "I am going to create the following plan for using my sleep thinking systematically."

_____

_____

_____

_____

Sleep Thinking Prompt: "Another night of sleep thinking. How lovely!"

_____

_____

_____

_____

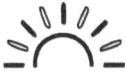

Morning Processing:

_____

_____

_____

_____

_____

_____

_____

_____

_____

75

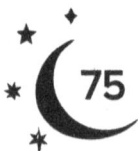

A NEW WAY TO THINK

"You must master a new way to think before
you can master a new way to be."
—MARIANNE WILLIAMSON

Sleep thinking is a "new way to think." It may be as old as the species, but it may be new to you. You always had those billions of neurons at the ready, waiting to sleep think at your behest. But did anyone ever invite you to use them in that way? That is my invitation to you. Employ your full capabilities to meet life. The brilliant, free resource of sleep thinking will not let you down.

Journal Prompt: "The following is my plan for using my brain's natural ability to think while I sleep."

_____

_____

_____

_____

Sleep Thinking Prompt: "I wonder what my sleep thinking will deliver tonight."

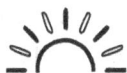

_____

_____

_____

_____

Morning Processing:

_____

_____

_____

_____

_____

_____

_____

_____

_____

Epilogue

Problems of every sort confront us daily. Those that we can't solve produce ongoing stress. The problem might be at work, it might be with a child, it might be with a creative project, it might be with some global, shared problem like war, authoritarianism, or climate disaster. Each of these wears us down.

For some of these, we require clarity and action steps. For others, we more need serenity and acceptance. All of them, the actionable and the intractable, benefit from the application of your best brain, that brain that wants to serve you as you sleep. Freed of its daily occupations, all those billions of neurons are there for you, ready to help.

The process I've described is easy to understand. You relax into sleep, guiding your brain with a sleep thinking prompt that you offer your brain lightly. The prompt aims your neurons where you would like them to go. You surrender to the night, you sleep well, and, in the morning, you remember to check in with yourself to see what you brain has to offer.

This is a brilliant but not foolproof process. The answer you are seeking may take a long time in coming. Some famous math problems have proven unsolvable for centuries! As great a mathematician as you may be, as many neurons as you may have at your disposal, you may still not be able to solve the Reimann hypothesis or the

P-vs-NP problem. We understand that problems of all sorts, whether personal, practical, creative, scientific, or global, can prove intractable.

But many can be solved! The problem that you are currently facing may be one of those. Consider that it is. Be positive and optimistic. That positivity and optimism will help the process. If you're saying to yourself, "I can't possibly solve this," you're giving your mind the message, "Don't bother." And it won't. It'll think about something else. Don't invite your brain to distract itself and go elsewhere. Stay positive, hopeful, and focused.

Do you have a clear picture of two of the acts of your three-act play, but not the third? Sleep thinking is perfect for that. Do you have some big concerns about your current career path? Invite your brain to sleep on your next steps. Are you troubled by your lack of control, about how you can't change the person you live with or the world? Create a sleep thinking prompt that invites your brain to plot a course that takes such realities into account.

What might that sound like? Maybe, "How can I gain some control in my life?" or "How can I live peacefully in my exact circumstances?" Start to get practiced at creating sleep thinking prompts that really speak to your brain, that clearly communicate what you're after. Creating clear, on-point prompts is a lovely part of the practice of self-awareness. Actionable prompts are the fruit of a conversation you have with yourself about how best to live your life.

Let me end with an anecdote about a client of mine I'll call Mary. Mary needed help raising money for the documentary film she dearly wanted to make. Thinking about all the options available to her, including the many crowdfunding ones, confused and exhausted her. I invited her to sleep on it, and her second night's sleep thinking produced the following "answer": "Talk to your mother."

Mary had completely forgotten that her mother was connected in that world! How can such forgetfulness possibly happen? But it can and it does, all the time. We got to examine why Mary had blocked that knowledge from her waking brain, that her mother was there to help. It turned out that there were many reasons why she had blocked that knowledge, and they were real and significant. But by airing them, it became clear that they were significant, but not insurmountable.

Mary went to her mother for help—and the film got made. Like Mary, you too may discover that the answers you get from sleep thinking may force you to look at what's really going on. Let that be okay. Be brave. You want those answers, even if they make difficulties for you or bring up painful material. Just stewing will hurt you emotionally and physically. Better to get answers and deal with the fruits of your sleep thinking.

My hope is that you will enjoy the sleep thinking process, be served by it, and make use of it as your primary resource for solving problems of all sorts. It is free, and it is what your brain really wants to do. Your brain would love to serve you, if you will invite it, aim it, and listen to it. Good night to you— and, tomorrow morning, may you discover that you've been gifted with exactly the information you were looking for.

About Eric Maisel

Eric Maisel is an internationally-recognized diplomat coach, the author of 60+ books in the areas of coaching, creativity, life purpose, meaning, and mental health, and President of the International Association of Creative and Performing Artists.

A retired family therapist and active master coach, Dr. Maisel is the lead editor for the Ethics International Press Critical Psychology and Critical Psychiatry series, which takes a critical look at the current mental disorder paradigm and the influence of psychiatry on society's institutions. Its 2026 offerings are *Artists in Crisis* and *Existential Wellness*.

His popular *Psychology Today* blog "Rethinking Mental Health" has more than 3.5 million views, and, in conjunction with Noble-Manhattan Coaching, he has developed three training programs, a Creativity Coach Certificate Program, an Existential Wellness Coach Certificate Program, and a Relationship Coach Certificate Program.

Dr. Maisel regularly blogs for The Good Men Project and Fine Art America, presents sponsored workshops, webinars, and keynotes, and maintains an international coaching practice. He has been interviewed more than five hundred times on the topics of coaching, creativity, life purpose, meaning and mental health.

Among his 60+ titles are *Brave New Mind* (January, 2026), *Night Brilliance* (February, 2026), *Existential Wellness Coaching* (September, 2026), *Choose Your Life Purposes*, *Parents Who Bully*, *Redesign Your Mind*, *Rethinking Depression*, *Coaching the Artist Within*, *Why Smart People Hurt*, *The Coach's Way*, *Fearless Creating*, *The Future of Mental Health*, *The Power of Daily Practice* and *The Van Gogh Blues.*

Dr. Maisel has delivered his five-day Deep Writing workshop at conference centers like the Omega Institute, Esalen, Hollyhock, the Kripalu Yoga & Retreat Center, and the Art of Living Retreat Center; and in locales like San Francisco, New York, Dublin, Prague, London, Rome, and Paris. His weekly blogs include "The Craft of Coaching with Eric Maisel" and "Tales of the Creative Life."

Dr. Maisel was born in the Bronx, grew up in Brooklyn, and attended Manhattan's Stuyvesant High School. Among his degrees are a B.S. in Philosophy from the University of Oregon and a B.A. in Psychology, a M.A. in Creative Writing, and an M.S. in Counseling, all from San Francisco State University. A retired California licensed marriage and family therapist, he lives in Walnut Creek, California with Ann Mathesius Maisel, his wife of forty-eight years.

Please visit Dr. Maisel at https://www.ericmaisel.com or contact him at ericmaisel@hotmail.com

Connect with Me!

I'd love to stay in touch with you and hear your thoughts, questions, comments, and stories. I welcome all reader feedback. Please be in touch!

Here are some of the ways you can connect with me:

- Email me: ericmaisel@hotmail.com

- Visit my website: https://ericmaisel.com/

- Post a review on Amazon, Goodreads, or wherever you buy and read books. Every reader review helps make books like this one more accessible to others.

- Subscribe to my newsletter. It arrives twice a week and alerts you to my latest books, workshops, and other offerings. And you get a lovely free gift for subscribing! Visit here to subscribe: https://ericmaisel.com/newsletter/

- Subscribe to my Substack. I post new pieces every week, about the artist's life, meaning and purpose, coaching, and the many other things that interest me. Visit here to subscribe: https://maiselthinkingaloud.substack.com/

- If you're interested in better understanding the current "mental disorder" landscape, I invite you to look at the Ethics International Press Critical Psychology and Critical Psychiatry series of books, for which I am the lead editor. See current volumes in the series here: https://ericmaisel.com/ethics-international-press/

- If you're an arts organization, a creative or performing artist (a writer, painter, actor, musician, filmmaker, etc.), someone interested in the creative life, or someone with a loved one in the arts, please take a look at the International Association of Creative and Performing Artists, where I serve as President. You can learn more here: https://iacpa.global/

- Check out my other books. There are more than 60 of them! Take a look here: https://ericmaisel.com/books/

Please stay in touch!

BOOKS BY ERIC MAISEL

Nonfiction

20 Communication Tips for Families

20 Communication Tips at Work

60 Innovative Cognitive Strategies for the Bright, the Sensitive and the Creative

A Writer's Paris

A Writer's San Francisco

A Writer's Space

Affirmations for Artists (reissued, 2026)

Become a Creativity Coach Now!

Brainstorm

Brave New Mind (forthcoming, 2026)

Coaching the Artist Within

Choose Your Life Purposes

Creative Recovery (with Susan Raeburn)

Creativity for Life

Deep Writing

Everyday You

Existential Wellness Coaching (forthcoming, 2026)

Fearless Creating (reissued, 2026)

Helping Parents of Diagnosed, Distressed and Different Children

Helping Survivors of Authoritarian Parents, Siblings and Partners

Humane Helping

Life Purpose Boot Camp

Lighting the Way

Living the Writer's Life

Making Your Creative Mark

Mastering Creative Anxiety

Overcoming Your Difficult Family

Parents Who Bully

Performance Anxiety

Redesign Your Mind

Rethinking Depression

Secrets of a Creativity Coach

Ten Zen Seconds

The Art of the Book Proposal

The Atheist's Way

The Creativity Book

The Coach's Way

The Future of Mental Health

The Life Purpose Diet

The Magic of Sleep Thinking

The Power of Daily Practice

The Van Gogh Blues

Toxic Criticism

Unleashing the Artist Within

What Would Your Character Do?

Why Smart, Creative and Highly Sensitive People Hurt

Why Smart People Hurt

Why Smart Teens Hurt

Write Mind

Your Great Coaching Career

Fiction

Aster Lynn

Dismay

Murder in Berlin

The Black Narc (as Jeffrey Feinman)

The Blackbirds of Mulhouse

The Fretful Dancer

The Kingston Papers (as R. S. Silverman)

The Pen

Settled

Journals and Sketchbooks

Affirmations for Self-Love (with Lynda Monk)

Artists Speak

Night Brilliance

Why Smart People Hurt Journal

Writers and Artists on Devotion

Writers and Artists on Love

Edited Collections

Artists in Crisis (forthcoming, 2026, with Susan Raeburn and Arnoldo Cantu)

Critiquing the Psychiatric Model (with Chuck Ruby)

Deconstructing ADHD

Existential Wellness (forthcoming, 2026, with Don Laird
    and Arnoldo Cantu)

Hearing Critical Voices

Humane Alternatives to the Psychiatric Model (with
    Chuck Ruby)

Inside Creativity Coaching

Institutionalized Madness (with Arnoldo Cantu and
    Chuck Ruby)

Practical Alternatives to the Psychiatric Model of Mental
    Illness (with Arnoldo Cantu and Chuck Ruby)

The Coach's Guide to Completing Creative Work (with
    Lynda Monk)

The Creativity Workbook for Coaches and Creatives

The Great Book of Journaling (with Lynda Monk)

Theoretical Alternatives to the Psychiatric Model of Mental
    Disorder Labeling (with Arnoldo Cantu and Chuck Ruby)

Transformational Journaling for Coaches, Therapists and
    Clients (with Lynda Monk)

Meditation Decks

Everyday Calm

Everyday Creative

Everyday Smart

Certification Programs

Creativity Coach Certification Program

Existential Wellness Coach Certification Program

Relationship Coach Certification Program

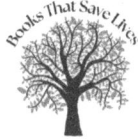

Books That Save Lives came into being in 2024 when the editor and publisher, Brenda Knight, heard directly from readers and authors that certain self-help, grief, psychology books, and journals were providing a lifeline for folks. We live in a stressful world where it is increasingly difficult not to feel overwhelmed, worried, depressed, and downright scared. We intend to offer support for the vulnerable, including people struggling with mental wellness and physical illness as well as people of color, queer and trans adults and teens, immigrants and anyone who needs encouragement and inspiration.

From first responders, military veterans, and retirees to LGBTQ+ teens and to those experiencing the shock of bereavement and loss, our books have saved lives. To us, there is no higher calling.

We would love to hear from you! Our readers are our most important resource; we value your input, suggestions, and ideas.

Please stay in touch with us and follow us at:

https://www.booksthatsavelives.net
https://www.instagram.com/booksthatsavelives/
https://www.facebook.com/people/Books-That-Save-Lives/
https://www.youtube.com/@BooksThatSaveLives

www.ingramcontent.com/pod-product-compliance
Lightning Source LLC
Chambersburg PA
CBHW011220290320
41931CB00044B/3463